Morgellons Disease
A Beginner's Quick Start Guide to Understanding and Managing the Condition
Patrick Marshwell

Copyright ©2024 by Patrick Marshwell

All rights reserved.

No portion of this book may be reproduced in any form without written permission from the publisher or author, except as permitted by U.S. copyright law.

mf

Contents

Disclaimer	1
Introduction	3
1. What is Morgellons Disease?	5
2. Why Diagnosing Morgellons is Difficult	11
3. Current Theories on Morgellons Causes	18
4. Relation to Conditions Such as Lyme Disease	25
5. Treatment and Management Techniques	34
6. Dietary Management for Morgellons Disease	42
7. Skin and Body Care for Managing Morgellons Disease	54
8. Resources for Caregivers	60
Conclusion	67
FAQs	72
Resources and Helpful Links	76

Disclaimer

By reading this disclaimer, you are accepting the terms of the disclaimer in full. If you disagree with this disclaimer, please do not read the guide.

All of the content within this guide is provided for inform- ational and educational purposes only, and should not be accepted as independent medical or other professional advice. The author is not a doctor, physician, nurse, mental health provider, or registered nutritionist/dietician. Therefore, using and reading this guide does not establish any form of a physician-patient relationship.

Always consult with a physician or another qualified health provider with any issues or questions you might have regarding any sort of medical condition. Do not ever dis- regard any qualified professional medical advice or delay seeking that advice because of anything you have read in this guide. The information in this guide is not intended to be any sort of medical advice and should not be used in lieu of any medical advice by a licensed and qualified medical pro- fessional.

The information in this guide has been compiled from a variety of known sources. However, the author cannot attest to or guarantee the accuracy of each source and thus should not be held liable for any errors or omissions.

You acknowledge that the publisher of this guide will not be held liable for any loss or damage of any kind incurred as a result of this guide or the reliance on any information provided within this guide. You acknowledge and agree that you assume all risk and responsibility for any action you undertake in response to the information in this guide.

Using this guide does not guarantee any particular result (e.g., weight loss or a cure). By reading this guide, you acknow- ledge that there are no guarantees to any specific outcome or results you can expect.

All product names, diet plans, or names used in this guide are for identification purposes only and are the property of their respective owners. The use of these names does not imply endorsement. All other trademarks cited herein are the property of their respective owners.

Where applicable, this guide is not intended to be a substitute for the original work of this diet plan and is, at most, a supplement to the original work for this diet plan and never a direct substitute. This guide is a personal expression of the facts of that diet plan.

Where applicable, persons shown in the cover images are stock photography models and the publisher has obtained the rights to use the images through license agreements with third-party stock image companies.

Introduction

Understanding Morgellon disease can be challenging, whether you've come across its complexities in medical discussions or through personal experiences. Navigating through countless questions without clear answers often leaves you searching for reliable resources. This comprehensive exploration is crafted to offer insights and support, serving as a beacon to guide you through the murky waters of Morgellons.

You might wonder why this resource is essential for you. Morgellons, an enigmatic condition, often leaves individuals feeling isolated and overlooked. The aim here is to provide a supportive companion that helps unravel the confusion and mystery surrounding it. By engaging with this material, you open doors to knowledge and empowerment, allowing for informed choices about your health and well-being.

In this guide, we will talk about the following;

- What is Morgellons Disease?
- Why Diagnosing Morgellons is Difficult
- Current Theories on Morgellons Causes

- Relation to Conditions Such as Lyme Disease

- Treatment and Management Techniques

- Dietary Management for Morgellons Disease

- Skin and Body Care for Managing Morgellons Disease

- Resources for Caregivers

Keep reading to learn more about how this valuable resource can empower you with deeper insights. Each page is a step towards clarity, helping you to face the challenges that Morgellons may present with confidence and understanding. By the end of this guide, you'll not only have a grasp of what Morgellons is but also know how to manage it effectively.

Chapter 1
What is Morgellons Disease?

Morgellons disease is a mysterious condition that has puzzled both patients and medical professionals. People with Morgellons report experiencing crawling sensations on or under the skin, and they often find thread-like fibers emerging from skin sores.

These symptoms can be quite distressing, leading to significant discomfort and impacting daily life. Despite the vivid experiences of those affected, Morgellons is not officially recognized as a distinct disease by many health authorities, which adds to the complexity of understanding this condition.

Historical Context and Discovery

Morgellons disease first came to widespread attention in the early 2000s. It was named by Mary Leitao, a mother whose son exhibited unusual skin symptoms that she struggled to find answers for in conventional medical diagnoses.

She named the condition after a similar skin disorder described in France several centuries earlier. Since then, Morgellons has been the subject of various studies and research efforts aimed at uncovering its origins and characteristics. Despite these efforts, clear answers remain elusive, contributing to ongoing debates within the medical community.

The Controversy Surrounding Morgellons

The controversy surrounding Morgellons disease largely stems from differing opinions on its nature and cause. Many medical professionals view it as a psychosomatic condition, similar to other disorders where physical symptoms are believed to stem from emotional or mental stress. This perspective suggests that the fibers seen by patients may be external contaminants or a result of compulsive skin picking.

On the other hand, patients and some researchers advocate for a deeper exploration of potential biological causes, such as bacterial or environmental factors. This divide has created tension between patients seeking validation and treatment, and a medical community that often lacks clear diagnostic criteria and consensus.

The lack of conclusive research and a standardized approach to diagnosis contributes to the ongoing debate and frustration for those affected by Morgellons. For individuals experiencing the symptoms, the quest for understanding and relief continues, often requiring a combination of medical guidance and personal management strategies.

Common Symptoms of Morgellons Disease

Morgellons disease presents a puzzling array of symptoms that deeply affect patients' lives, highlighting the complexity and challenges in understanding and managing this condition.

1. **Skin Sensations:** Patients frequently report sensations of crawling, biting, or stinging on or under the skin. These sensations can be intense and persistent, often described as feeling like insects moving on the skin, which can lead to significant discomfort and distress.

2. **Appearance of Fibers:** A hallmark symptom of Morgellons is the appearance of unusual thread-like fibers or granules that seem to emerge from the skin. These fibers can vary in color, including blue, red, black, or white, and are often found in or around skin sores.

3. **Skin Sores:** The condition is also characterized by persistent skin sores that may arise from repeated scratching due to the intense itching and discomfort. These sores can be painful, slow to heal, and are prone to infection, further complicating the patient's condition.

4. **Fatigue:** Many individuals with Morgellons experience chronic fatigue, a deep-seated tiredness that daily rest doesn't alleviate. This fatigue can impact daily activities and reduce overall quality of life, making it challenging for patients to maintain normal routines.

5. **Joint Pain:** Patients often report experiencing joint pain, which can range from mild discomfort to more severe aches.

This symptom can exacerbate feelings of fatigue and contribute to difficulties in maintaining physical activity.

6. **Cognitive Difficulties:** Cognitive issues, such as memory problems and trouble concentrating, are also common among those with Morgellons. These difficulties can affect work, learning, and social interactions, adding to the stress and frustration experienced by patients.

These symptoms collectively create a challenging condition for patients, impacting both physical and mental health. Understanding and managing these symptoms with a healthcare provider's guidance is crucial for improving the quality of life for those affected by Morgellons disease.

Diagnosis Process for Morgellons Disease

Diagnosing Morgellons disease is a complex and often challenging process for healthcare providers due to the lack of standardized criteria. Here's how medical professionals typically approach the diagnosis:

1. **Initial Examination:** The process begins with a thorough physical examination to assess the patient's symptoms and overall health. Healthcare providers pay close attention to the skin, looking for sores and fibers, and take note of the patient's descriptions of skin sensations.

2. **Medical History:** A detailed medical history is crucial for ruling out other conditions that share similar symptoms,

such as skin infections, dermatitis, or parasitic infestations. Understanding the patient's past health issues and any psychological factors is essential for a holistic approach.

3. **Skin Biopsies and Fiber Analysis:** Skin biopsies may be conducted to examine the tissues under a microscope, looking for any abnormalities. Fiber analysis can also be performed to identify the nature of the fibers reported by patients. However, results often indicate that these fibers are external contaminants, making it difficult to establish a direct link to Morgellons.

4. **Psychological Evaluations:** Considering the controversial nature of Morgellons, some healthcare providers evaluate the psychological aspects, exploring whether the symptoms might be related to mental health conditions like stress or anxiety. This approach helps in providing comprehensive care that addresses both physical and mental health needs.

5. **Challenges and Complexities:** The diagnosis of Morgellons remains controversial due to the lack of clear diagnostic markers and the overlap with other medical and psychological conditions. This ambiguity can lead to frustration for both patients and healthcare providers, as the path to understanding and managing Morgellons often requires a multifaceted and individualized approach.

Healthcare providers work closely with patients to manage symptoms and improve quality of life, even when a definitive diagnosis remains elusive. Collaboration between patients and medical professionals is key to navigating the complexities of Morgellons disease.

Chapter 2
Why Diagnosing Morgellons is Difficult

Diagnosing Morgellons disease is a complex process, fraught with challenges that stem from a lack of standardized tests and the symptom overlap with other conditions. These factors create a diagnostic landscape that is both intricate and often frustrating for patients and healthcare providers alike.

Lack of Standard Tests

The challenge of diagnosing Morgellons disease primarily stems from the absence of definitive diagnostic tests and standardized criteria. This situation places healthcare providers in a difficult position, as they lack the clear protocols typically available for diagnosing other conditions. Consequently, they must rely heavily on clinical observation and patient-reported symptoms.

This reliance can introduce variability and subjectivity into the diagnostic process, as patients may describe their experiences differently, and healthcare providers may interpret symptoms based on their own clinical expertise.

1. **Impact on Diagnostic Process**

The lack of standard tests means that diagnosing Morgellons often becomes a process of elimination. Healthcare providers must systematically rule out other potential conditions that could explain the patient's symptoms.

This can include a wide range of dermatological issues, such as eczema or psoriasis, as well as other medical conditions that present with similar symptoms. This method can be time-consuming and requires a thorough investigation of the patient's medical history and current health status.

1. Implications for Patient Care

The absence of clear diagnostic criteria can have significant implications for patient care. Without a definitive diagnosis, patients may experience feelings of frustration and distress. They might feel that their symptoms are being dismissed or misunderstood by the medical community, leading to a strained patient-provider relationship. This experience can be emotionally taxing and might exacerbate their symptoms or lead to a sense of isolation.

Additionally, the uncertainty surrounding the diagnosis can delay the initiation of effective treatment plans. Patients may be left without appropriate symptom management strategies, potentially worsening their quality of life. This highlights the need for healthcare providers to offer empathetic support and reassurance, while actively engaging in finding the most suitable management approach for each patient.

1. Necessity of Ruling Out Other Conditions

The diagnostic process for Morgellons involves the careful exclusion of other conditions that share similar clinical features. This requires a comprehensive approach that takes into account various possibilities, such as skin disorders, infections, and psychological factors.

The complexities involved in this differential diagnosis underscore the importance of a multidisciplinary approach. Collaborating across specialties can help ensure that all potential causes are considered and addressed, ultimately leading to more accurate diagnosis and effective care for patients experiencing Morgellons disease.

Overlap with Other Conditions

Diagnosing Morgellons disease is further complicated by the symptom overlap with other medical and psychological conditions. This overlap creates significant challenges for healthcare providers trying to distinguish Morgellons from other ailments that present similar clinical features.

1. Dermatological Disorders

Many symptoms of Morgellons, such as skin sores, itching, and the sensation of crawling or stinging, are also common in dermatological conditions like eczema and psoriasis. These skin disorders can cause severe discomfort and visible skin changes, making it difficult to differentiate them from Morgellons without a detailed examination.

Additionally, conditions like scabies or other parasitic infections can produce similar sensations and skin manifestations, adding layers to the diagnostic puzzle.

1. **Psychological Issues**

Psychological factors can also play a role in the presentation of Morgellons symptoms. Stress and anxiety, for instance, can exacerbate sensations of itching or crawling, leading to increased skin picking and resulting sores.

Some symptoms might be psychosomatic, where psychological distress manifests as physical symptoms, complicating the diagnostic process further. This overlap with psychological issues requires healthcare providers to consider mental health assessments as part of their diagnostic approach.

1. **Challenges in Differentiation**

The similarity in symptoms across various conditions necessitates a careful and comprehensive approach to diagnosis. Healthcare providers must distinguish between Morgellons and other potential diagnoses through thorough patient history, clinical examinations, and sometimes by consulting various specialists. This comprehensive approach ensures that all possibilities are considered and that the patient receives appropriate care.

1. **Multidisciplinary Approach**

Given these complexities, a multidisciplinary approach is crucial. Collaborating across specialties such as dermatology, psychiatry, and infectious diseases ensures a holistic understanding of the patient's condition.

This collaboration is vital for ruling out other potential causes and providing more accurate diagnoses. By integrating insights from different fields, healthcare providers can develop more effective and tailored management strategies for patients presenting with Morgellons-like symptoms.

Ultimately, the overlap with other conditions emphasizes the need for ongoing research and education among healthcare providers to improve diagnostic accuracy and ensure effective patient care.

Comprehensive and Individualized Approach

Addressing the complexities of Morgellons disease requires a comprehensive and individualized approach, essential for managing this challenging condition. Given the intricate nature of its symptoms, healthcare providers often need to engage in cross-specialty collaboration to fully address both the physical and mental health aspects involved.

1. Importance of Multidisciplinary Collaboration

The symptoms of Morgellons can span across dermatological, psychological, and even infectious domains. Therefore, collaboration among dermatologists, psychiatrists, infectious disease specialists, and other healthcare professionals is crucial.

Each specialist brings a unique perspective that can contribute to a more complete understanding of the patient's condition. This collaborative approach ensures that no aspect of the patient's health is overlooked, leading to a more thorough evaluation and management plan.

1. Effective Management Despite Diagnostic Challenges

Even when a definitive diagnosis remains elusive, a multidisciplinary strategy can significantly aid in the effective management of symptoms. By pooling expertise, healthcare teams can create comprehensive care plans tailored to each patient's unique needs.

This approach often involves not only medical treatments but also supportive therapies, such as counseling or stress management techniques, which can help alleviate the psychological burden of the disease.

1. Benefits of Personalized Care Plans

Personalized care plans are at the heart of an individualized approach. These plans take into account the specific symptoms, lifestyle, and preferences of each patient, ensuring that care is both relevant and efficient. Such customization can improve patient adherence to treatment and enhance overall outcomes, providing patients with a greater sense of control and agency over their health.

1. Role of Ongoing Research

Ongoing research plays a pivotal role in refining diagnostic and management approaches for Morgellons. By continually exploring new insights into the potential causes and mechanisms of the disease, researchers can contribute to the development of more precise diagnostic tools and effective treatments. This research not only aids in improving the immediate care for current patients but also lays the groundwork for future advancements that could lead to a clearer understanding of Morgellons.

Ultimately, this comprehensive and individualized approach underscores the importance of seeing each patient as a whole, addressing both the physiological and psychological dimensions of their experience. Through collaboration, personalized care, and ongoing research, healthcare providers strive to offer the best possible support to those living with Morgellons disease.

Ongoing research efforts aim to improve the understanding and diagnosis of Morgellons. Scientists are exploring potential genetic, environmental, and infectious factors that might contribute to the condition, hoping to develop more precise diagnostic tools. These research initiatives are crucial for moving towards a future where Morgellons can be diagnosed more effectively, leading to better outcomes for those affected.

While the road to a clear diagnosis remains challenging, these efforts underscore the dedication of the medical community to unraveling the mysteries of Morgellons disease. By continuing to investigate the condition's complexities, healthcare providers aim to offer clearer answers and more compassionate care to those living with Morgellons.

Chapter 3

Current Theories on Morgellons Causes

Understanding Morgellons disease is a complex endeavor, with multiple theories and ongoing debates about its origins. These theories span from biological to psychological, and even environmental aspects, highlighting the intricate nature of the condition.

Bacterial and Parasitic Theories

The idea that Morgellons may have bacterial or parasitic origins is one of the more debated theories in understanding this mysterious condition. Here's a closer look at the arguments and evidence supporting this line of thought.

1. Borrelia and Lyme Disease Connection

A significant focus within this theory is the potential involvement of Borrelia, a type of bacteria linked to Lyme disease. Many individuals diagnosed with Morgellons also report symptoms consistent with Lyme disease, suggesting a possible connection between the two.

Some researchers hypothesize that Borrelia might play a role in the development of Morgellons, potentially influencing the skin manifestations and other symptoms observed in patients. This hypothesis is intriguing, especially given the reported overlap in clinical presentations between Morgellons and Lyme disease.

1. Bacterial DNA in Skin Lesions

Another piece of supporting evidence comes from the detection of bacterial DNA in the fibers extracted from Morgellons skin lesions. These fibers have been found to contain traces of DNA from various bacteria, including those related to Borrelia.

This finding bolsters the theory that Morgellons might have an infectious component, suggesting that the fibers could be a result of bacterial activity or interactions within the skin. However, the origins and significance of these fibers remain subjects of scientific investigation, and more research is needed to understand their exact nature and role.

1. Controversies and Challenges

Despite these intriguing observations, the theory of bacterial or parasitic involvement in Morgellons is not without controversy. Critics point out the lack of consistent, concrete scientific evidence directly linking Morgellons to a specific bacterial or parasitic cause. The presence of bacterial DNA in skin lesions could be incidental or unrelated to the primary condition, indicating that further studies are necessary to establish causality.

Need for Further Research

The ongoing debate underscores the need for more comprehensive research to clarify the potential role of bacteria or parasites in

Morgellons disease. Rigorous scientific exploration is essential to determine whether these findings are coincidental or indicative of a deeper, underlying biological process.

By advancing our understanding through dedicated research efforts, we can aim to resolve these controversies and improve diagnostic and treatment strategies for those affected by Morgellons.

Psychological Theories

Exploring Morgellons disease through the lens of psychological theories presents a different perspective on what might contribute to the symptoms experienced by patients. This approach focuses on the potential role of mental health factors in the manifestation and perception of symptoms.

1. Delusional Parasitosis and Symptom Manifestation

Some researchers suggest that the symptoms of Morgellons might originate from psychological conditions, such as Delusional Parasitosis. This condition involves a mistaken belief of being infested with parasites, which can lead individuals to experience intense skin sensations like crawling, stinging, or biting.

These sensations might result in scratching and skin sores, which are commonly reported by Morgellons patients. This theory posits that psychological distress or underlying mental health disorders could be at the root of these physical symptoms, and addressing these mental health issues might provide relief.

1. The Role of Mental Health in Symptom Perception

Mental health plays a crucial role in how symptoms are perceived and experienced. Psychological stress, anxiety, and depression can intensify the perception of physical sensations, leading to a heightened awareness and sensitivity to bodily changes.

For individuals with Morgellons, this means that psychological factors could amplify the severity and persistence of their symptoms, creating a cycle of discomfort and distress.

1. Mixed Reactions and Patient Perspectives

While the psychological theory offers insights into potential contributors to Morgellons symptoms, it is met with mixed reactions. Many patients are apprehensive about this explanation, feeling that it invalidates their experiences and dismisses the physical aspects of their condition.

They might worry that a psychological label could lead to stigmatization or inadequate care. This highlights the importance of approaching Morgellons with empathy and understanding, acknowledging both the physical and psychological components of the disease.

1. Importance of a Holistic Approach

Considering psychological factors is critical in adopting a holistic approach to diagnosing and treating Morgellons. Mental health should be integrated into the overall care strategy, ensuring that patients receive comprehensive support that addresses both their physical symptoms and psychological well-being.

This balanced approach can help healthcare providers offer more effective and compassionate care, acknowledging the complexity of Morgellons and the diverse factors that influence it. By valuing patients' perspectives and incorporating mental health into treatment plans, we can work towards more personalized and patient-centered care.

Environmental Factors

The theory that environmental factors could contribute to Morgellons disease is gaining attention as researchers try to understand the origins of this perplexing condition. Here's a deeper look into how certain environmental agents might influence Morgellons symptoms.

1. Environmental Agents and Symptom Triggers

Some theories propose that exposure to specific chemicals or pollutants could trigger or worsen Morgellons symptoms. These environmental agents include pesticides, industrial chemicals, and heavy metals, which have been scrutinized for their potential impact on health.

The rationale for investigating these substances lies in their known ability to cause skin irritations and other health issues, leading some to believe that they could be linked to the mysterious symptoms of Morgellons.

1. Reports from Individuals with Morgellons

Many individuals with Morgellons report that their symptoms began or worsened after exposure to certain environmental factors. For example, some claim that their symptoms started following pesticide use or after moving to areas with high industrial activity.

These anecdotal accounts suggest a possible connection between environmental exposure and the onset of Morgellons symptoms, prompting further research into this area.

1. Current State of Research

Despite growing interest, research into the environmental factors associated with Morgellons is still in its early stages. While several studies have been conducted, a definitive link between specific environmental agents and Morgellons has yet to be established.

The complexity of isolating environmental variables and their interactions with biological systems makes this a challenging area of study. Researchers emphasize the need for rigorous investigations to confirm whether these factors play a significant role in Morgellons.

1. Implications for Prevention and Treatment

If a connection between environmental factors and Morgellons is established, it could have important implications for prevention and treatment strategies. Identifying specific triggers could lead to the development of guidelines to help individuals avoid exposure to harmful agents. Additionally, understanding the role of environmental factors could inform treatment approaches, potentially leading to new interventions that address both environmental and physiological aspects of the disease.

As research progresses, the hope is to uncover more concrete evidence that can guide healthcare providers and patients in managing Morgellons effectively. Until then, a multidisciplinary approach that considers both environmental and other potential causes remains key in addressing this complex condition.

Chapter 4
Relation to Conditions Such as Lyme Disease

When examining Morgellons disease, it's essential to consider its connection to other conditions, notably Lyme Disease. Both Morgellons and Lyme Disease present a puzzling array of symptoms that often overlap, making diagnosis and treatment challenging.

Symptom Overlap Between Morgellons and Lyme Disease

The overlap in symptoms between Morgellons disease and Lyme disease presents a significant challenge for both patients and healthcare providers. These conditions share a range of persistent physical, psychological, and neurological symptoms that can greatly affect daily life. These commonalities not only complicate the diagnostic process but also highlight the critical need for careful clinical evaluation and a better understanding of both diseases.

1. Shared Symptoms and Their Impact on Daily Life

One noticeable similarity between Morgellons and Lyme disease is debilitating fatigue, which goes far beyond normal tiredness. It can make basic tasks like cooking or walking seem impossible. This chronic fatigue often isolates individuals as they struggle to maintain relationships or pursue professional goals.

Joint pain is another significant symptom of both conditions. This pain can vary from a mild ache to severe discomfort that affects mobility, making it hard to grip objects or perform tasks requiring fine motor skills. Over time, this constant pain can lead to frustration, helplessness, and even mental health issues like depression or anxiety.

Neurological symptoms are common in both diseases. Patients often report cognitive issues like memory problems and difficulty concentrating, known as "brain fog." These issues can disrupt clear thinking, organization, or problem-solving, affecting work and personal life. Mood changes, including irritability and sudden emotional shifts, are also common. These symptoms can make it difficult for individuals to advocate for themselves in medical settings, as they might struggle to explain symptoms clearly.

1. **Challenges in Diagnosing Morgellons and Lyme Disease**

The shared symptoms of Morgellons and Lyme disease create challenges for accurate diagnosis. Symptoms like fatigue, joint pain, and cognitive issues are common in many illnesses, including fibromyalgia, chronic fatigue syndrome, multiple sclerosis, and mental health disorders like depression.

This overlap often leads to misdiagnosis or delayed diagnosis, delaying appropriate treatment. For example, a patient with joint pain and fatigue might first be diagnosed with a rheumatological condition instead of Lyme or Morgellons. Similarly, neurological symptoms might be attributed to stress or anxiety, especially if tests don't show clear issues. For Morgellons patients, the situation is even more complex due to ongoing debate in the medical community about its classification.

1. Broader Implications for Patients and Providers

This diagnostic complexity has far-reaching consequences. For patients, the delay in getting an accurate diagnosis can result in prolonged suffering and worsening symptoms. They may feel disbelieved or dismissed, particularly if their symptoms fall outside of what is understood in conventional medical frameworks. This can lead to a deterioration in trust between patients and healthcare providers.

For healthcare professionals, the challenge lies in distinguishing between these two conditions while taking into account the broader differential diagnoses. Both Morgellons and Lyme disease require detailed patient histories, thorough physical examinations, and sometimes repeated testing to reach a reliable conclusion. However, even these steps are not always sufficient, as no single test can definitively rule out or confirm either condition in all cases.

1. The Importance of Accurate Diagnosis

Accurate diagnosis is essential for effective treatment. Although Morgellons and Lyme disease share symptoms, their treatments differ. Lyme disease is usually treated with antibiotics, while Morgellons treatments vary and are often debated. Misdiagnosis can lead to ineffective or even harmful treatments.

Understanding their symptom overlap can help research the causes of these diseases and develop targeted therapies. This can improve outcomes for individuals with either condition.

For those with Morgellons and Lyme disease, diagnosis and treatment can be frustrating. The symptom overlap complicates their medical journey, requiring persistence from patients and expertise from healthcare providers. Enhanced awareness, ongoing research, and open communication between patients and doctors are crucial to improving care.

Co-Infections in Morgellons and Lyme Disease

The relationship between Morgellons and Lyme disease is already complex, but the potential for co-infections adds another layer of difficulty. A co-infection occurs when a person is infected with multiple pathogens at the same time.

This is particularly common with Lyme disease, as the same ticks that carry Borrelia burgdorferi—the primary bacteria responsible for Lyme—often also transmit other harmful microorganisms. These additional infections can amplify symptoms, blur the diagnostic lines, and challenge the effectiveness of treatment strategies.

1. **Understanding Co-Infections and Their Role in Disease**

When someone develops a co-infection, their immune system is forced to combat multiple pathogens simultaneously. Unfortunately, each of these pathogens can produce its own set of symptoms or worsen existing ones. This overlap often results in a more severe and prolonged illness compared to a single infection. For instance, a patient with both Lyme disease and a co-infection like Babesia or Bartonella may experience heightened levels of fatigue, persistent fever, or more severe neurological issues.

The presence of co-infections can also hinder the body's response to treatment. Certain pathogens have mechanisms for evading or suppressing the immune system, making it even more difficult for the body to recover fully. Additionally, standard antibiotic regimens prescribed for Lyme disease may not be sufficient to address co-infections, leaving patients with unresolved symptoms even after treatment.

1. Common Co-Infections in Lyme Disease

Ticks are not exclusively hosts for Borrelia burgdorferi. They are reservoirs for a wide variety of infectious agents, including bacteria, protozoa, and viruses. Two of the most commonly reported co-infections in Lyme disease are caused by Babesia and Bartonella, but others like Anaplasma and Ehrlichia may also complicate the picture.

- **Babesia:** This pathogen is a parasite that infects red blood cells, causing a condition similar to malaria called babesiosis. Symptoms of Babesia can include fever, chills, night sweats, and significant fatigue. Because it attacks blood cells,

Babesia infections are often associated with symptoms like shortness of breath and anemia, which may not initially seem related to Lyme disease.

- **Bartonella:** Often referred to as "cat scratch disease" when contracted from cat scratches or bites, Bartonella can also be transmitted through tick bites. This bacterium is notorious for causing skin lesions, severe headaches, and neurological disturbances. Patients with Bartonella frequently report amplified anxiety and mood fluctuations, alongside physical symptoms like swollen lymph nodes and chronic pain.

Both Babesia and Bartonella can magnify the discomforts already associated with Lyme disease, making symptoms more debilitating and recovery more elusive.

1. Challenges in Diagnosing Co-Infections

Pinpointing co-infections presents a formidable challenge for healthcare providers. One major issue lies in the significant overlap of symptoms between Lyme disease, Morgellons, and these additional infections. For instance, fatigue and cognitive issues might be attributed to Lyme disease, while the true underlying cause—Babesia or Bartonella—goes undiagnosed and untreated.

Further complicating matters is the fact that standard diagnostic tests for Lyme may not detect co-infections. Many of these infections require their own specialized testing, which is not always performed unless specifically requested. Babesia, for example, often necessitates a blood smear or PCR (polymerase chain reaction) testing for detection. Bartonella testing can be even more problematic, as the bacteria tend to cause persistent low-level infections that may not readily show up in blood tests.

1. The Complexity of Treating Co-Infections

Treating co-infections requires a tailored approach. A course of antibiotics designed to target Borrelia burgdorferi may have little to no effect on Babesia, which requires anti-malarial drugs, or Bartonella, which might need different classes of antibiotics. Additionally, the presence of multiple pathogens can lead to increased inflammation and immune dysfunction, making the body less responsive to treatment overall.

Patients with Morgellons and Lyme disease who also have co-infections may require prolonged or combination therapies. For many, this involves a mix of antimicrobial medications, immune-supportive treatments, and symptom management strategies. However, finding the right balance can be a painstaking process involving trial and error, which contributes to the frustration experienced by both patients and clinicians.

1. The Importance of Comprehensive Testing and Personalized Care

Given the multi-faceted challenges posed by co-infections, the importance of comprehensive diagnostic testing cannot be overstated. Healthcare providers must approach cases of Lyme disease, Morgellons, and associated co-infections with a holistic perspective, considering the possibility of multiple underlying infections. Incorporating specialized tests into the diagnostic process can help identify co-infections early, allowing for more targeted treatment.

Equally critical is the need for personalized care plans that address the unique combination of infections and symptoms experienced by each patient. This often requires collaboration among specialists, including infectious disease experts, rheumatologists, and neurologists, to ensure a comprehensive approach to diagnosis and treatment.

Co-infections significantly complicate the clinical picture of Morgellons and Lyme disease, adding to the suffering of patients and the pressures on healthcare providers. These overlapping conditions require heightened awareness, advanced diagnostic techniques, and individually tailored treatment strategies to achieve the best possible outcomes. By acknowledging and addressing the role of co-infections, the medical community can take a crucial step toward improving the care and recovery for those grappling with these complex conditions.

Implications for Patient Care

Co-infections have major implications for patient care, highlighting the need for thorough testing to identify all possible infections for an accurate diagnosis. Once infections are pinpointed, healthcare providers can craft personalized treatment plans targeting each specific infection and its symptoms. This customized approach is essential for managing the complex interaction of symptoms and enhancing patient outcomes.

Understanding the connections between Morgellons, Lyme Disease, and other co-infections is vital for advancing patient care and guiding future research. Recognizing shared symptoms and potential co-infections can lead to better diagnostic tools and treatment strategies, ultimately offering hope for those affected by these elusive conditions.

By continuing to explore these connections, researchers and healthcare providers can work towards more effective solutions and a deeper understanding of the underlying causes of these diseases.

Chapter 5
Treatment and Management Techniques

Addressing Morgellons disease involves a multifaceted approach to manage symptoms and improving the quality of life for those affected. Here's an exploration of effective symptom management and available medical interventions.

Symptom Management

Effective symptom management is essential for individuals with Morgellons disease to maintain daily functioning, improve overall well-being, and enhance their quality of life. By adopting a multifaceted approach, patients can address both physical and emotional challenges associated with this condition. Below are detailed strategies organized into distinct sections:

1. **Lifestyle Changes**

Making thoughtful changes to one's lifestyle can significantly impact health and energy levels:

- **Balanced Diet**: A nutritious diet ensures the body gets essential nutrients to function well. Eating fruits, vegetables, lean proteins, and whole grains can boost energy, strengthen immunity, and aid healing. Foods rich in antioxidants and vitamins may also reduce inflammation, helping manage fatigue and joint pain.

- **Regular Exercise**: Adding physical activity to daily routines offers both physical and mental benefits. Activities like walking, swimming, or yoga improve cardiovascular health, reduce stiffness, and increase flexibility. Exercise releases endorphins, acting as natural mood boosters, and helps reduce stress and depression often experienced by Morgellons patients.

1. **Stress Management Techniques**

Stress often exacerbates the symptoms of Morgellons. Developing methods to manage stress is crucial to symptom control and mental health:

- **Mindfulness Meditation**: Practicing mindfulness helps focus on the present, reducing anxiety and creating calm and clarity to better manage symptoms.

- **Yoga**: Combining postures, breathing, and meditation, yoga offers a holistic way to relieve stress while building strength and flexibility.

- **Deep-Breathing Exercises**: Techniques like slow diaphragmatic breathing quickly reduce anxiety and promote relaxation, with just a few minutes a day lowering stress levels.

1. **Supportive Therapies**

Supportive therapies address the emotional and mental health aspects of Morgellons, which are often as debilitating as the physical symptoms:

- **Cognitive-Behavioral Therapy (CBT)**: This therapy helps patients identify and change negative thought patterns, aiding in coping with mood changes, depression, and cognitive challenges linked to Morgellons, while building mental resilience.

- **Support Groups**: Connecting with others facing similar challenges reduces isolation and offers support. These groups provide a safe space for sharing experiences and encouragement, which is therapeutic.

- **Art or Music Therapy**: Expressive therapies use creativity to help individuals process emotions in non-verbal ways, especially beneficial for patients who find it hard to express their struggles.

By integrating these strategies into a personalized care plan, patients can create a foundation for better symptom management. Each approach works in harmony to address different aspects of Morgellons disease, empowering individuals to regain control over their health and improve their quality of life.

Medical Interventions

Medical treatments play a critical role in addressing the symptoms and potential underlying causes of Morgellons disease. While there is no universally accepted treatment protocol, targeted medical interventions can offer relief and improve patients' quality of life.

1. **Antibiotics**

Antibiotics are often a first-line treatment, particularly in cases where co-existing bacterial infections, such as those associated with **Lyme Disease**, are suspected. Morgellons disease has been linked to Lyme Disease in numerous cases, and addressing the bacterial component can be crucial for symptom relief.

- **Purpose and Function**: Antibiotics help to reduce the bacterial load in the body, potentially alleviating symptoms like chronic joint pain, fatigue, and neurological dysfunction. By targeting bacterial infections, these medications may also indirectly help reduce inflammation caused by the immune system's response to pathogens.

- **Examples**: Common antibiotics used for Lyme and other bacterial infections include doxycycline, cefuroxime, or amoxicillin, depending on the severity of the infection and the patient's response.

- **Considerations**: Long-term antibiotic use can lead to side effects such as stomach upset, antibiotic resistance, or altered gut flora. Frequent monitoring by a healthcare provider is essential to balance the benefits with potential risks during prolonged treatment.

1. **Antiparasitic Treatments**

Antiparasitic medications are considered in cases where Morgellons symptoms are suspected to be linked to parasitic infections, though their effectiveness in Morgellons disease remains a topic of debate.

- **Purpose and Target**: These treatments aim to eliminate possible parasitic involvement, which could be exacerbating symptoms like skin irritation, lesions, or sensations of crawling or itching. Antiparasitic agents work by targeting parasites that may contribute to the disease, even in cases where clear evidence of infestation is absent.

- **Medications Given**: Medications like ivermectin or albendazole are sometimes prescribed. These drugs aim to combat parasitic organisms thought to live in or on the skin.

- **Challenges and Limitations**: The lack of conclusive evidence linking parasites directly to Morgellons makes this approach controversial. Misuse or overuse of antiparasitic drugs can also result in side effects, unnecessary toxicity, or exacerbation of underlying skin or neurological symptoms.

1. **Other Medical Interventions**

While less commonly discussed, additional medical treatments may be explored in managing Morgellons symptoms. These therapies focus on symptom relief rather than addressing potential causes.

- **Topical Treatments**: Anti-inflammatory creams, antifungal ointments, or soothing skin preparations may be used to address lesions, itching, or discomfort. These provide localized relief and help promote healing in damaged skin.

- **Neurological Symptom Management**: For patients experiencing cognitive or neurological challenges, medications like low-dose antidepressants, anticonvulsants (e.g., gabapentin or pregabalin), or anti-anxiety drugs may be considered to manage associated symptoms like pain, anxiety, or sleep disturbances.

- **Pain Management**: Chronic pain, particularly in the joints or muscles, can be managed with over-the-counter pain relievers like acetaminophen or NSAIDs. More severe cases may benefit from prescription-strength medications tailored to the patient's needs.

Integrating Medical Interventions into a Treatment Plan

To maximize the effectiveness of medical interventions, it is vital to integrate them into a **comprehensive, patient-centered treatment plan**:

- **Personalized Approach**: No two Morgellons cases are identical, and symptoms can vary significantly from one patient to another. Tailoring medical treatments to suit individual needs ensures a higher chance of success.

- **Collaborative Care**: Healthcare providers should work closely with patients to assess the impact of treatments, adjust dosages, and explore alternative options when required. This partnership is essential given the variable and often puzzling nature of the disease.

- **Monitoring and Flexibility**: Regular follow-ups are necessary to avoid adverse effects and evaluate the progress of treatments. Addressing any changes in symptom presentation is key to a flexible treatment approach, which can adapt as new challenges arise.

By understanding the potential benefits and limitations of antibiotics, antiparasitic treatments, and other medical options, healthcare providers can create a well-rounded plan aimed at alleviating both the physical and emotional burdens of Morgellons disease. With careful oversight and a focus on individualized care, these interventions offer hope for improved outcomes and a higher quality of life for patients.

Comprehensive Treatment Plans

A successful approach to treating Morgellons involves combining symptom management with medical interventions in a comprehensive treatment plan. Personalized care is vital, as each patient's experience with Morgellons can vary widely. Healthcare providers play a key role in tailoring treatments to meet individual patient needs, ensuring that all aspects of the disease are addressed.

Challenges and Considerations

Treating Morgellons presents several challenges, including the lack of consensus on its origins and the variability of symptoms among patients. This variability necessitates a flexible and adaptable treatment approach, where healthcare providers must balance addressing immediate symptoms with considering potential underlying causes.

Ultimately, a patient-centered approach that integrates both lifestyle and medical interventions offers the best chance for improving outcomes. By understanding the complexities of Morgellons, healthcare providers can deliver more effective and compassionate care, helping patients manage this elusive and often misunderstood condition.

Chapter 6
Dietary Management for Morgellons Disease

Dietary management plays a crucial role in supporting overall health and managing symptoms for individuals with Morgellons disease. While proper nutrition alone cannot cure the condition, it can strengthen the body, enhance the immune system, and help alleviate some of the associated discomforts. Below is a detailed overview of nutritional support and specific dietary recommendations that may be beneficial:

Importance of Nutritional Support and a Balanced Diet

A balanced diet is essential for maintaining energy levels, boosting immunity, and promoting the body's natural healing processes. For individuals with Morgellons, whose symptoms may include chronic fatigue, skin lesions, and cognitive difficulties, proper nutrition can help mitigate the strain on the body and improve overall well-being.

- **Immune System Support:** A strong immune system is vital for fighting off potential co-infections, such as those associated with Lyme Disease, and for maintaining skin health. A diet rich in vitamins, minerals, and antioxidants can help the body combat inflammation and oxidative stress, both of which may exacerbate Morgellons symptoms.

- **Tissue Repair and Skin Healing**: Nutrients like protein, vitamin C, and zinc are instrumental in tissue repair and skin regeneration, making them essential for patients dealing with persistent lesions or open wounds.

- **Cognitive and Energy Support**: Symptoms like brain fog and low energy levels may be alleviated through stable blood sugar levels and adequate consumption of brain-healthy nutrients, such as omega-3 fatty acids and B vitamins.

A balanced diet that includes plenty of fruits, vegetables, lean proteins, and healthy fats can provide the necessary nutrients for supporting the body's natural healing processes and managing Morgellons symptoms.

Specific Dietary Recommendations

While there is no specific "Morgellons Diet," certain dietary recommendations may be beneficial to individuals dealing with this condition. It is always best to consult with a healthcare professional before making significant changes to your diet, especially if you are on any medications or have existing medical conditions.

1. Anti-Inflammatory Foods

- **Fatty Fish**: These are rich in omega-3 fatty acids, which are essential for reducing inflammation. Omega-3s help decrease the production of inflammatory molecules and are crucial for brain health. Regular consumption of fatty fish like salmon and mackerel can help maintain a balanced inflammatory response, potentially easing skin irritation and other symptoms associated with Morgellons.

- **Nuts and Seeds**: Walnuts, chia seeds, and flaxseeds are not only high in omega-3s but also contain fiber and protein, making them a great addition to any diet. They help reduce inflammation and support heart health. Including these in your diet can provide a steady source of energy and essential nutrients.

- **Olive Oil**: Known for its heart-healthy benefits, extra virgin olive oil contains oleocanthal, which has anti-inflammatory properties similar to non-steroidal anti-inflammatory drugs (NSAIDs). Using olive oil as a primary fat source can help reduce inflammation and improve cardiovascular health.

- **Turmeric**: This spice is renowned for its anti-inflammatory and antioxidant properties, primarily due to curcumin. Curcumin can help reduce inflammation at the molecular level. Adding turmeric to your diet, especially when combined with black pepper to enhance absorption, can support joint health and reduce chronic inflammation.

- **Leafy Greens**: These are packed with vitamins, minerals, and antioxidants. Vitamin E, found in leafy greens, plays a key role in protecting the body from pro-inflammatory molecules. Incorporating a variety of greens into your meals can boost your immune system and help manage inflammation.

1. **High-Fiber Foods**

- **Whole Grains**: Foods like oats and quinoa are excellent sources of dietary fiber, which is crucial for digestive health. Fiber helps regulate the digestive system, prevent constipation, and maintain a healthy weight. Whole grains also provide essential nutrients like B vitamins and iron.

- **Fruits**: High in fiber, fruits like apples and berries also provide vitamins and antioxidants. The fiber in fruits helps slow digestion, providing a gradual release of energy and keeping you full longer. This can help stabilize blood sugar levels and support weight management.

- **Vegetables**: Vegetables such as broccoli and Brussels sprouts are rich in fiber and essential nutrients. They support digestive health and provide antioxidants that help fight inflammation. Including a variety of vegetables in your diet ensures you get a wide range of nutrients.

- **Legumes**: Lentils and chickpeas are not only high in fiber but also provide plant-based protein. They help maintain healthy blood sugar levels and support heart health. Legumes are versatile and can be used in soups, salads, and stews.

1. **Probiotic-Rich Foods**

- **Yogurt**: A great source of probiotics, yogurt helps maintain a healthy balance of gut bacteria. This can improve digestion and boost the immune system. Choosing plain, unsweetened yogurt ensures you avoid added sugars that can disrupt gut health.

- **Kefir**: This fermented milk drink is rich in probiotics and often easier to digest than regular milk. Kefir can improve gut health and enhance the body's ability to absorb nutrients. It's a versatile ingredient that can be used in smoothies or consumed on its own.

- **Fermented Foods**: Foods like sauerkraut and kimchi are rich in probiotics and enzymes that support digestion. They can help balance gut bacteria and improve nutrient absorption. Including fermented foods in your diet can enhance gut health and support the immune system.

- **Prebiotic Foods**: Foods like garlic and onions feed beneficial gut bacteria, helping probiotics thrive. Prebiotics are essential for maintaining a healthy gut microbiome, which is crucial for overall health and well-being.

1. **Antioxidant-Rich Foods**

- **Berries**: These fruits are packed with antioxidants like anthocyanins, which help reduce inflammation and protect against oxidative stress. Berries are also high in fiber and vitamin C, supporting immune health and skin repair.

- **Dark, Leafy Greens**: Rich in vitamins A, C, and E, these greens provide antioxidants that protect cells from damage. They support immune function and help maintain healthy skin.

- **Nuts and Seeds**: Almonds and sunflower seeds are high in vitamin E and selenium, which have antioxidant properties. These nutrients help protect the skin and reduce inflammation.

- **Green Tea**: Known for its high content of polyphenols like EGCG, green tea has powerful antioxidant and anti-inflammatory effects. Regular consumption can support heart health and improve skin resilience.

- **Bright Vegetables**: Vegetables like carrots and sweet potatoes are high in beta-carotene, which the body converts to vitamin A. This nutrient is essential for skin health and immune function.

By focusing on these food groups, you can create a diet that supports overall health, reduces inflammation, and helps manage symptoms associated with Morgellons disease. Always consult with a healthcare provider before making significant dietary changes to ensure they are appropriate for your individual health needs.

Foods to Avoid for Managing Morgellons Disease

When dealing with Morgellons symptoms, it's important to focus on a clean, nutrient-dense diet while avoiding certain foods that could worsen inflammation, disrupt gut health, or weaken the immune system. Below is a guide on foods and beverages to limit or eliminate and the reasons why avoiding them might help manage symptoms and support overall well-being.

1. Processed Foods

Processed foods are often loaded with added sugars, unhealthy fats, additives, and preservatives that can trigger inflammation and impair your body's natural detoxification processes. Chronic inflammation is commonly associated with worsening skin conditions and can potentially intensify Morgellons symptoms such as skin discomfort or irritation.

Examples to Avoid: Packaged snacks like chips, cookies, and candies; frozen meals; sugary breakfast cereals; fast food; and processed meats like sausages, hot dogs, or bacon.

Why They're Problematic:

- **Added Sugars** directly fuel inflammation in the body and can feed harmful gut bacteria, upsetting the balance of your microbiome.

- **Trans Fats and Hydrogenated Oils**, often found in processed baked goods and margarine, are notorious for causing cellular inflammation.

- **Artificial Colors and Flavors** may irritate sensitive systems and lead to allergic or inflammatory responses in some individuals.

- **What to Do Instead**: Opt for whole, minimally processed foods whenever possible. Swap sugary snacks with fresh fruit or nuts, and make simple recipes at home using fresh ingredients.

1. Gluten and Dairy

Though not universally problematic, gluten and dairy products are known to cause inflammation or digestive issues in some people, particularly those with sensitivities, intolerances, or autoimmune tendencies. Many individuals managing Morgellons symptoms have reported improvements after cutting out these food groups, possibly due to reduced systemic irritation or improved digestive health.

Examples to Avoid:

- For **Gluten**: Foods made from wheat, rye, and barley, such as bread, pasta, cereals, and baked goods.

- For **Dairy**: Milk, cheese, butter, cream, and yogurt (unless lactose-free or plant-based alternatives).

Why They're Problematic:

- **Gluten** can damage the intestinal lining and promote inflammation in those with gluten sensitivity or celiac disease. A weakened gut barrier may exacerbate immune system imbalances.

- **Dairy** contains lactose and casein proteins, which may be difficult to digest and inflammatory for some people. Dairy is also linked to acne and other skin issues in some cases.

What to Do Instead:

Replace gluten-containing foods with alternatives like quinoa, brown rice, or gluten-free bread and pasta.

Opt for non-dairy milk alternatives such as almond milk, coconut milk, or oat milk, and experiment with plant-based cheeses or yogurt substitutes.

1. **Caffeine**

While caffeine is a natural stimulant and can have some benefits when consumed in moderation, it can also contribute to anxiety, poor sleep, and heightened skin sensitivity in some individuals, especially if consumed in excess. Since many Morgellons patients report heightened sensations or discomfort, reducing caffeine may help the nervous system regulate better.

Examples to Avoid:

Coffee, energy drinks, sodas, and certain types of tea with high caffeine levels (e.g., black tea).

Why It's Problematic:

- **Stimulant Effects** can heighten restlessness and stress, potentially exacerbating skin sensations like itching or crawling feelings.

- **Sleep Disruption** caused by caffeine may hinder the body's ability to repair and regenerate, worsening symptoms over time.

- **Gut Irritation** can occur with high caffeine intake, affecting digestion and microbiome balance.

What to Do Instead:

Choose caffeine-free herbal teas like chamomile, peppermint, or rooibos. If you prefer coffee, consider decaf options.

1. **Alcohol**

Alcohol consumption can suppress immune function, disrupt digestion, and further inflame the body, making it particularly important to limit or avoid for those managing chronic conditions. Even moderate drinking can impair the body's ability to heal skin lesions or maintain energy levels, which are often areas of concern for people with Morgellons disease.

Examples to Avoid: Beer, wine, spirits (e.g., vodka, rum, whiskey), and cocktails.

Why It's Problematic:

- **Toxin Build-Up** occurs because the liver prioritizes processing alcohol, delaying other toxin removal processes, which could worsen symptoms.

- **Dehydration** caused by alcohol can dry out skin and aggravate skin lesions or irritation.

- **Sugar Content** found in cocktails and sweetened drinks can contribute to systemic inflammation and upset gut health.

What to Do Instead:

Drink plenty of water and herbal teas to stay hydrated. You can also try creating alcohol-free "mocktails" with seltzer, fresh fruit, and herbs for a refreshing alternative.

By avoiding or minimizing these foods and beverages, you reduce the potential triggers for inflammation, gut imbalance, and immune suppression. This dietary approach may not cure Morgellons but can help you better manage symptoms and feel more in control of your overall health. Always consult with a healthcare practitioner to create a plan tailored to your unique needs.

Supplements to Support Symptom Management

While managing your diet is crucial in managing Morgellons symptoms, certain supplements may also help support your body's immune system and overall health. Here are a few examples of supplements that have shown promise in helping manage Morgellons disease:

1. **Probiotics**: Probiotics can help restore balance to the gut microbiome, which is often disrupted in people with chronic conditions like Morgellons disease. Look for strains such as Lactobacillus acidophilus or Bifidobacterium lactis.

2. **Vitamin D**: Vitamin D plays an essential role in maintain-

ing a healthy immune system and has been shown to improve symptoms of autoimmune diseases. As many people with Morgellons disease also have underlying autoimmune conditions, supplementing with vitamin D may be beneficial.

3. **Omega-3 fatty acids**: Omega-3s have anti-inflammatory properties and can help reduce inflammation in the body. Look for a high-quality fish oil supplement or incorporate foods rich in omega-3s, such as salmon, into your diet.

4. **Zinc**: Zinc is an important mineral that supports immune function and wound healing. People with Morgellons disease often experience slow wound healing, so supplementing with zinc may help speed up this process.

Again, it's essential to consult with a healthcare practitioner before adding any supplements to your regimen, as they can interact with medications and may not be suitable for everyone. Additionally, taking supplements alone will not cure Morgellons disease, but they may help alleviate symptoms and support overall health.

Chapter 7
Skin and Body Care for Managing Morgellons Disease

Individuals living with Morgellons disease often face unique challenges related to skin discomfort and irritation. Establishing a gentle and supportive skin and body care routine can be an essential part of symptom management and overall well-being. Below are practical tips and recommendations to help maintain healthy skin and alleviate discomfort.

Skin Care Routines: Tips for Maintaining Skin Health

Following a dedicated skincare routine can help protect your skin, soothe irritation, and support healing. These practices are designed to minimize any further damage and improve skin resilience.

1. **Gentle Cleansing**

- Use a mild, fragrance-free cleanser that's designed for sensitive skin. Harsh soaps or strong detergents can strip the skin of its natural oils, exacerbating dryness and irritation.

- Avoid scrubbing or using abrasive tools on your skin, as this can cause micro-damage and worsen symptoms.

- Wash your face and affected areas with lukewarm water.

Hot water can dry out or irritate sensitive skin.

Benefits: Gentle cleansing removes dirt, oil, and potential irritants while preserving the skin's moisture barrier, reducing irritation and itching.

1. Moisturizing

- Apply a thick, fragrance-free moisturizer immediately after cleansing while the skin is still damp. This locks in hydration and soothes dry, irritated skin.

- Opt for moisturizers containing ingredients like ceramides, hyaluronic acid, or aloe vera, which can calm and protect the skin.

- For areas prone to irritation or lesions, you can use healing ointments like petroleum jelly or products with colloidal oatmeal.

Benefits: Regular moisturizing softens the skin, relieves dryness, and supports barrier repair, which is crucial for minimizing the discomfort of skin lesions.

1. Applying Protective Products

- Consider using barrier creams or ointments on areas prone to friction or constant irritation. These can act as a shield against further damage or external irritants.

- Sunscreen is essential if skin is exposed to sunlight—choose a broad-spectrum sunscreen with SPF 30 or higher that is free of fragrances and harsh chemicals.

Benefits: Protective products help shield the skin from harmful elements, maintain its integrity, and promote healing over time.

1. Targeted Care for Lesions

- Do not pick at or scratch lesions, as this can lead to infection, scarring, or prolonged healing.

- Use antiseptic sprays or ointments to keep areas of broken skin clean and reduce the risk of infection.

- Consult a healthcare provider for specific medicated creams or treatments that may alleviate irritation or promote faster healing of wounds.

Benefits: Focused care on affected areas minimizes the risk of complications like infection and helps speed up recovery.

1. Avoiding Irritants

- Steer clear of harsh exfoliants, alcohol-based products, and strong chemical treatments, as they can further inflame or irritate the skin.

- Use hypoallergenic laundry detergents and avoid fabric softeners that may leave residues on clothes and trigger reactions.

Benefits: Reducing your exposure to irritants lowers the likelihood of skin inflammation or aggravation.

Hygiene Practices: Daily Practices to Alleviate Discomfort

Hygiene is incredibly important for alleviating discomfort and preventing complications like secondary infections. Developing daily habits can make a significant difference in how you manage your symptoms.

1. Regular Bathing

- Bathe daily using lukewarm water and a gentle, sulfate-free body wash. Avoid using strongly fragranced soaps, as they may irritate sensitive skin.

- Add Epsom salts or colloidal oatmeal to your bath for soothing relief from itching or irritation.

- Limit bath time to 10–15 minutes to prevent the skin from drying out.

Benefits: Consistent bathing keeps the skin clean, improves comfort, and reduces the buildup of irritants that might worsen symptoms.

1. Using Hypoallergenic Products

- Opt for products labeled as hypoallergenic, dermatologically tested, and free of potential irritants like parabens, sulfates, and dyes.

- Choose natural, mild deodorants and soaps that are designed for sensitive skin.

Benefits: Using hypoallergenic products ensures that your skin is less likely to react adversely, helping to maintain healthy, calm skin.

1. **Maintaining a Clean Environment**

- Wash bed linens and clothing frequently in hot water to remove potential allergens, irritants, or debris.

- Use mattress and pillow protectors made from allergy-friendly materials for extra cleanliness.

- Regularly vacuum or clean your living space to reduce dust mites, fibers, or particles that may irritate the skin.

Benefits: A clean environment reduces the exposure to irritants that can trigger discomfort or worsen skin issues.

1. **Proper Nail Care**

- Keep your nails trimmed and clean to avoid causing unintentional scrapes or damage when scratching.

- For individuals prone to scratching at night, consider wearing gloves to prevent injury to the skin.

Benefits: Proper nail hygiene minimizes the chance of skin infections caused by bacteria or dirt under the nails.

1. **Comfortable Clothing**

- Wear loose-fitting, breathable fabrics such as cotton to avoid friction and excessive heat against the skin.

- Avoid rough, synthetic materials like wool or polyester, which can exacerbate irritation.

Benefits: Comfortable clothing prevents chafing, overheating, and unnecessary aggravation of sensitive or damaged skin.

1. **Hydration**

- Drink plenty of water throughout the day to keep your skin and body hydrated from the inside out.

- Use a humidifier in your living space to add moisture to the air, especially in dry environments or during winter months.

Benefits: Proper hydration supports the skin's natural healing processes, keeping it supple and less prone to irritation.

By adopting a combination of effective skin care routines and thoughtful hygiene practices, you can better manage the challenges of Morgellons disease. These habits not only reduce discomfort and irritation but also promote healing and improve overall skin health. While these recommendations are supportive, it's important to seek guidance from a healthcare provider to ensure they align with your specific needs and symptoms.

Chapter 8

Resources for Caregivers

Caring for someone with Morgellons can be both rewarding and challenging. In this chapter, we will explore some helpful resources for caregivers to support the well-being of their loved ones.

Support Networks

Connecting with others who understand the challenges of caregiving can make a huge difference. Here are some resources to help you find support:

1. **Online Communities**

   - **Morgellons Support Groups on Facebook** Many private groups are dedicated to Morgellons caregivers and patients. These communities offer a safe space to share experiences, ask for advice, and feel understood. Search for "Morgellons support" on Facebook to find groups.

   - **Morgellons Disease Awareness (MDA)** The MDA is an organization that often hosts online forums and webinars for patients and caregivers. Their website also includes lists of worldwide support resources.

1. **Local Support Groups**

- Check with local hospitals, community centers, or churches for caregiver support groups or chronic illness-focused meetings.

- **The National Alliance for Caregiving (NAC)** While not specific to Morgellons, the NAC provides a wealth of national resources and connections for caregivers.

1. **Professional Counseling**

Caregiving can be emotionally demanding. Speaking to a therapist or counselor who specializes in caregiving or chronic illness can help you handle stress and improve your emotional resilience.

Remember, being part of a support network reassures you that you're not alone in this experience.

Educational Materials

Understanding Morgellons is key to providing effective care. These resources can guide you in learning more about the condition and addressing its complex challenges.

1. **Books**

- *Morgellons - The Skin and the Brain Connection* by Cindy Casey Holman This book dives into Morgellons' physical and neurological impacts, offering insights for caregivers and patients alike.

- *The Caregiver's Survival Handbook* by Alexis Abramson- While not specific to Morgellons, this resource offers strategies for managing caregiver stress and navigating the caregiving role.

1. **Articles & Research**

- Look up articles from medical journals that discuss Morgellons, such as studies published by the International Lyme and Associated Diseases Society (ILADS).

- Websites like **ScienceDirect** or **PubMed** can provide peer-reviewed research on Morgellons' symptoms and treatments.

1. **Online Resources**

- **The Charles E. Holman Morgellons Disease Foundation (CEHMDF)** This organization is a hub of educational materials, scientific studies, and advocacy updates for the Morgellons community.

- **Mayo Clinic** Though not Morgellons specific, their caregiving guidance section provides practical advice for caregivers managing chronic illnesses.

Continued learning can empower you to feel more confident and capable in your caregiving role.

Caregiving Tips

Providing care for someone with Morgellons requires patience, empathy, and adaptability. Here are some strategies for daily routines, symptom management, and maintaining well-being.

Daily Care Routines

1. **Create a Structured Routine:** Establish consistent daily habits to help the individual feel a sense of stability. Include time for meals, medication, rest, and skin care.

2. **Assist with Hygiene and Skin Care:** Since skin lesions are a primary symptom of Morgellons, help the individual maintain good hygiene to prevent infections:

    - Use mild, fragrance-free cleansers and moisturizers.
    - Encourage gentle cleaning of lesions to avoid irritation.
    - Keep bandages clean and dry if needed.

3. **Encourage a Nutritious Diet and Hydration:** Boost their immunity and energy by providing balanced meals rich in fruits, vegetables, and lean proteins. Staying hydrated is equally vital.

Symptom Management

Caring for an individual with Morgellons can be challenging, but by utilizing available resources and adopting effective strategies, caregivers can significantly enhance the quality of life for those affected.

1. **Support Their Comfort:**

   - Provide clothing that's soft and non-irritating.
   - Consider air purifiers for a cleaner indoor environment if sensitivities exist.

2. **Monitor Medical Needs:**

   - Keep a notebook to track symptoms, medication schedules, and doctor visits. Bring this log to appointments to help healthcare providers understand patterns.

3. **Seek Professional Guidance:**

   - Work with doctors to address co-occurring conditions like anxiety, depression, or fatigue.
   - Ensure proper wound care if lesions require medical attention.

Supporting Their Emotional Well-being

Dealing with Morgellons can feel isolating and overwhelming for the individual you're caring for. Here's how you can support them emotionally:

- **Listen and Validate Their Feelings:** Even if you don't fully understand their experience, showing empathy can strengthen your bond.
- **Engage in Relaxing Activities:** Explore calming hobbies

together, such as painting, listening to music, or spending time outdoors.

- **Encourage Professional Support:** Encourage counseling or therapy for your loved one if they face mental health challenges.

<u>Taking Care of Yourself</u>

1. **Set Boundaries:** It's okay to say no to additional demands that will overextend you. Your well-being matters too.

2. **Take Breaks:** Regularly schedule time for yourself – whether it's a walk, reading a book, or calling a friend. Respite care services can provide temporary relief so you can recharge.

3. **Practice Self-Compassion:** Accept that you won't be "perfect" every day. Focus on doing your best and finding small moments of joy.

4. **Get Support When Needed:** Lean on your support network or seek professional help if you're struggling with burnout.

Caregiving is a marathon, not a sprint. Taking time to care for yourself ultimately helps you be a better caregiver.

Caring for someone with Morgellons can test your resilience, but it also opens the door to deep connection and understanding. By educating yourself, finding support, and practicing self-care, you can make a positive impact on your loved one's life while maintaining your own well-being. You are not alone in this; help and resources are available to guide you every step of the way.

Conclusion

Thank you for taking the time to explore this comprehensive guide on Morgellons disease. We know this wasn't a light read, and we deeply appreciate your commitment to understanding this complex and often misunderstood condition. Whether you're someone experiencing Morgellons directly, a caregiver, or simply looking to learn more, your willingness to educate yourself is a powerful step toward compassion, awareness, and positive change.

After reading this guide, you now have a clearer picture of what Morgellons disease is and why it presents such unique challenges. You've learned about its symptoms, its controversial nature, and the difficulties in receiving a diagnosis. Armed with this knowledge, you're better equipped to recognize the complexities of this condition and take meaningful steps for either your own health or the support of someone you love.

Morgellons is not a one-size-fits-all condition. Each person's experience is shaped by unique symptoms, emotional impacts, and even interactions with the healthcare system. This can feel overwhelming at times, particularly given the lack of definitive answers or universally recognized treatments. But what this guide shows you is that even amidst the uncertainty, there are ways to take control and actively manage the condition.

By now, you've seen that management boils down to a mix of awareness, self-care, and effective communication with healthcare providers. From creating tailored treatment plans to adopting healthier routines and improving your support network, there are practical tools at your disposal. Whether it's a simple change in diet, using gentle skin-care routines, or finding the right medical professional, every step you take is an act of resilience and self-empowerment.

Remember, Morgellons isn't just about the physical symptoms; it also affects your mental and emotional well-being. Luckily, with knowledge and a proactive mindset, you can address these challenges holistically.

One of the most important takeaways from this guide is that you're not helpless in the face of Morgellons. Understanding this condition—whether it's the theories about its causes, the overlap with other illnesses like Lyme disease, or the available treatment options—can make all the difference. Knowledge gives you power. It allows you to make informed decisions, advocate for yourself during doctor visits, and take charge of your own care.

If you're someone directly living with Morgellons, you've probably felt dismissed at times. Maybe you've even doubted yourself. This happens far too often with conditions that aren't widely understood. But remember, your experiences are valid. The fibers, the skin sensations, the fatigue, the cognitive struggles—they're real, and your effort to seek answers and find relief shows tremendous courage.

If you're a caregiver, pat yourself on the back for showing up. Supporting someone through a condition as complex as Morgellons isn't an easy task. Your willingness to care, learn, and adapt means the world to the person you're helping. Even if you don't have all the answers, your presence and patience are invaluable.

Living with Morgellons—or caring for someone who does—can sometimes feel like a lonely road. But the truth is, you are not alone. Others have walked this path and continue to find ways to thrive and take control of their well-being. Drawing from their stories can provide hope, perspective, and even inspiration to face tomorrow with fresh determination.

Your next step doesn't have to be monumental. Maybe it's committing to a small lifestyle change, like drinking more water or switching to hypoallergenic skin products. Maybe it's reaching out to a support group, finding a new healthcare provider, or scheduling that appointment you've been putting off. Each effort, no matter how minor it seems, represents progress.

And growth doesn't have to happen overnight. It's okay to take things one day at a time. Self-care, healing, and coping are ongoing journeys. Give yourself breathing room to process emotions, find strategies that work for you, and adjust when needed. Celebrate all your victories, big and small—they're proof that you're moving forward.

A key theme throughout this guide is the importance of community, both for individuals and caregivers. You don't need to do this alone. Find others who understand your challenges. Whether you join a local support group, participate in online discussions, or simply lean on friends and family, having people in your corner makes a world of difference.

If you're a caregiver, make sure you don't neglect your own needs. Burnout is real, and you're entitled to moments of rest, reflection, and rejuvenation. Strong caregivers remember the importance of self-care—not as a luxury but as a necessity for sustaining energy and compassion over the long haul. By taking care of yourself, you'll be better equipped to care for others.

Raising awareness about Morgellons is another powerful way you can contribute, whether you're a patient, caregiver, or ally. The more people know, the greater the understanding, empathy, and credibility this condition receives. Advocacy doesn't need to be on a grand scale. Simply sharing what you've learned with a friend or helping someone else find resources can amplify awareness and create ripples of change.

Remember, health and healing aren't confined to the physical realm. Acknowledgment and acceptance often begin within. Recognize your own strength and worth. You have the ability to face challenges head-on and adapt to life's uncertainties. Morgellons doesn't define you—your actions and determination do.

Before we part, we want to thank you once again for investing your time, effort, and attention to learn about Morgellons disease. This guide was designed to be a starting point—a resource to shine a light on a topic that too often gets left in the shadows. By reading through it, you've taken an important step that not only equips you with knowledge but also helps break the stigma surrounding this condition.

Your willingness to engage, empathize, and explore solutions is an encouragement to others. It's a sign of strength and resilience. Whether you're figuring out how to better manage the disease yourself or seeking ways to help someone else, every step forward matters. Every effort counts.

This is only the beginning of your journey. There's always more to learn and more opportunities to grow. Stay curious, stay hopeful, and keep moving forward at your own pace. The progress you make today forms the foundation for a brighter tomorrow.

Above all else, remember this truth—you are not alone in this. Others have faced Morgellons and found ways to reclaim joy, purpose, and fulfillment. There are resources, professionals, and communities ready to support you. By reaching out and staying determined, you'll find those connections and build the network of support you deserve.

Your story, your resilience, and your efforts matter. By empowering yourself with knowledge, engaging with the right resources, and cultivating empathy—for yourself and others—you're taking huge strides in navigating Morgellons with grace and courage.

Here's to your strength, your perseverance, and the better days ahead. Thank you for letting this guide be a part of your path.

FAQs

What is Morgellons disease, and why is it so controversial?

Morgellons disease is a perplexing condition where individuals report symptoms like crawling sensations on the skin, unusual fibers emerging from skin sores, and chronic fatigue. It's controversial because there is no consensus within the medical community on its cause. Some researchers attribute it to physical factors like bacterial infections, while others view it as a psychosomatic condition, leading to debates over its classification and treatment.

What are the common symptoms of Morgellons disease?

Key symptoms include:

- Crawling, stinging, or biting sensations on or under the skin.
- Fibers or thread-like substances emerging from skin lesions.
- Chronic skin sores that are slow to heal.

- Fatigue and joint pain.

- Cognitive difficulties like memory loss or "brain fog." These symptoms vary widely, making the condition challenging to diagnose and treat.

Why is diagnosing Morgellons so difficult?

Morgellons diagnosis is complicated due to the lack of standardized diagnostic criteria and symptom overlap with other conditions like eczema, Lyme disease, or psychological disorders. Doctors often rely on a process of elimination, ruling out other potential causes, which can be time-consuming and frustrating for patients. Additionally, the lack of consistent testing methods and differing opinions within the healthcare community add to the difficulty.

What treatment options are available for Morgellons disease?

There is no universal cure, but treatment focuses on symptom management:

- Antibiotics may be prescribed if co-infections like Lyme disease are suspected.

- Antiparasitic medications or topical treatments might be used for skin irritation.

- Supportive therapies, including stress management, cognitive-behavioral therapy (CBT), and counseling, can address emotional well-being.

- Lifestyle changes, such as a nutritious diet, regular exercise, and a strong emphasis on skin care, play a critical role in management.

How can dietary management help in Morgellons disease?

A balanced, anti-inflammatory diet can support overall health and symptom relief. Key dietary recommendations include:

- Consuming anti-inflammatory foods like fatty fish, leafy greens, and turmeric.

- Including probiotics (yogurt, kefir) and fiber-rich foods (whole grains, vegetables) to support gut health.

- Avoiding processed foods, excess sugar, caffeine, and alcohol that could worsen inflammation or disrupt the immune system. These nutritional strategies can enhance immune function and promote skin healing.

What skincare routines are helpful for managing Morgellons symptoms?

Gentle skincare is vital to soothe irritation and support healing:

- Use mild, fragrance-free cleansers and moisturizing creams with soothing agents like aloe vera or ceramides.

- Avoid scratching lesions to prevent infection.

- Apply protective creams or ointments to damaged areas and keep wounds clean with antiseptics.

- Wear loose, breathable cotton clothing and use hypoallergenic detergents. Practicing proper hygiene and maintaining consistent skin care can prevent further irritation and discomfort.

What resources are available for caregivers of individuals with Morgellons disease?

Caregivers can find support and information through:

- Online support groups and communities like Facebook's Morgellons forums.

- Organizations like the Charles E. Holman Morgellons Disease Foundation, providing education and advocacy.

- Books and articles to better understand the disease, like *Morgellons – The Skin and the Brain Connection* by Cindy Casey Holman.

- Professional counseling or caregiver support groups to manage emotional stress. Caregivers are encouraged to balance supporting their loved ones with self-care to avoid burnout.

Resources and Helpful Links

Seladi-Schulman, J., PhD. (2023, April 21). *Morgellons Disease.* Healthline. https://www.healthline.com/health/morgellons-disease

Dryden-Edwards, R., MD, & Mbbs, S. M. (2024, July 5). *Morgellons disease: Causes, symptoms, diagnosis & treatment.* MedicineNet. https://www.medicinenet.com/morgellons_disease/article.htm#:~:text=While%20there%20is%20no%20specific,like%20olanzapine%20or%20pimozide%2C%20respectively.

Delusional parasitosis. (n.d.). Mayo Clinic. https://www.mayoclinic.org/delusional-parasitosis/art-20044996

Ames, H. (2022, May 31). *Can diet help treat Lyme disease?* https://www.medicalnewstoday.com/articles/lyme-disease-diet

Can Morgellons Disease/Syndrome be linked to Lyme Disease? Where do the fibers come from that is embedded in a persons skin? Can this disease mimic the DNA of hair follicles that becomes very hard to remove from the given area? Why does. . . | Effective Health Care (EHC) Program. (n.d.). https://effectivehealthcare.ahrq.gov/get-involved/nominated-topic

s/can-morgellons-diseasesyndrome-be-linked-to-lyme-disease-where-do-the-fibers-come-from-that-is-embedded-in-a-persons-skin-can-this-disease-mimic-the-dna-of-hair-follicles-that-becomes-very-hard-to-remove-from-the-given-area-

Yuan, C., & Cohen, B. A., MD. (2022, October 27). Morgellons disease: a mysterious disease. *Dermatology Times.* https://www.dermatologytimes.com/view/morgellons-disease-a-mysterious-disease

Yan, B. Y., & Jorizzo, J. L. (2018). Management of Morgellons disease with Low-Dose Trifluoperazine. *JAMA Dermatology, 154*(2), 216. https://doi.org/10.1001/jamadermatol.2017.5175

www.ingramcontent.com/pod-product-compliance
Lightning Source LLC
LaVergne TN
LVHW052001060526
838201LV00059B/3773